the

PYRUVATE

phenomenon

the

PYRUVATE

phenomenon

❖ THE FACTS ❖
❖ THE BENEFITS ❖
❖ THE UNANSWERED QUESTIONS ❖

David Prokop

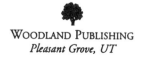

WOODLAND PUBLISHING
Pleasant Grove, UT

The information in this book is for educational purposes only and is not recommended as a means of diagnosing or treating an illness. All matters concerning physical and mental health should be supervised by a health practitioner knowledgeable in treating that particular condition. Neither the publisher nor author directly or indirectly dispense medical advice, nor do they prescribe any remedies or assume any responsibility for those who choose to treat themselves.

Contents

INTRODUCTION

It is the most talked about and exciting nutritional supplement to come along in years. Imagine a natural substance in our diet and our body which, if consumed in above normal amounts as a simple nutritional supplement, will produce a vast variety of health and fitness benefits.

Sounds too good to be true? Perhaps, but according to research studies that have been conducted thus far, there is reason to believe that this substance—pyruvate—may be one of the most beneficial and versatile food supplements ever developed. It has a list of benefits so broad it's doubtful if any other supplement can match it.

To be sure, there are some troubling questions still to be answered about pyruvate and its effectiveness, but in the highly competitive business of nutritional supplementation, it already seems to have grabbed the inside track on becoming a veritable dream supplement for a variety of interest groups:

- Athletes will presumably love pyruvate because it apparently increases exercise capacity (endurance), muscle energy and helps burn fat.[1]
- Dieters and others primarily looking to lose weight will love pyruvate because it helps people shed pounds and keep them off. The only question is how much pyruvate an individual needs to take.[2]
- Specifically health-conscious individuals—you know who you are!—will probably love pyruvate best of all because of its effectiveness in reducing cholesterol,[3] inhibiting free radical production,[4] defending against various diseases,[5] and even slowing the aging process itself.[6]

Significantly, these benefits have been substantiated by extensive research. Commercially available as a nutritional supplement only since early 1997, pyruvate has been studied for more than twenty-five years at major American universities, which makes it one of the most heavily researched nutritional supplements ever to hit the market. Since it is not a drug, pyruvate does not require FDA approval.

While pyruvate is not uncommon either in our diet or our body, the multiplicity of benefits that result from supplementing one's diet with pyruvate certainly are uncommon. The Congressional Dietary Supplement Act defines it simply as a nutritional supplement, but researchers and health experts are now referring to pyruvate as a nutraceutical, placing it in a category beyond that of a normal foodstuff or normal nutritional therapy.

When you bring into focus the whole picture that is emerging about pyruvate, it's clear that from a health standpoint it may potentially be the most valuable nutritional supplement of all. Not so much because of the sheer scope and variety of its benefits, but because research studies on animals have shown that pyruvate apparently prevents the formation of free radicals in the body—something no other substance, natural or otherwise, does as far as we know. Since free radicals have been implicated as the culprits in much of what goes wrong in our bodies—disease, aging, physical deterioration—the ramifications here are truly profound.

Some 735,000 Americans die of heart attacks each year; another 530,000 die of cancer.[7] The soaring cost of health care in America has reached truly stratospheric proportions; it's now in excess of 1.5 trillion dollars a year. Written numerically, that is $1,500,000,000,000, and to illustrate just how much money that is, if you were to spend a million dollars a day, it would take you more than 4000 *years* to spend 1.5 trillion dollars.

The obvious answer to the problems of illness and soaring health costs isn't more medicine, but more prevention—stopping disease before it begins. More research is needed on pyruvate and its free-radical connection, especially research involving humans rather than just animals. But what research has shown about pyruvate already is more than enough to pique the interest of any health-conscious person.

1

A REMARKABLE TESTAMENT

Pyruvate seemingly offers significant benefits for those at each end of the health or fitness spectrum, and everywhere in between—from the super fit on the one hand to the seriously health impaired on the other. Pax Beale of San Francisco, California, had the dubious privilege of experiencing both ends of the spectrum, and his story serves as a remarkable testament to pyruvate.

Beale has been a highly successful businessman (that's successful as in "millionaire") and a lifelong fitness enthusiast. His remarkable collection of achievements includes running across Death Valley to the top of Mt. Whitney, swimming from San Francisco to Alcatraz round trip at night, and racing an ocean liner on a bicycle to Alaska—and winning! He took up bodybuilding in his fifties after a back problem made it impossible for him to continue with his previous passion, distance running. He engaged in this new athletic interest with such zeal ("zeal" could be Beale's middle name) that he won the Mr. USA body-building championship at age sixty-one. He's been pumping iron ever since.

Now in his late sixties, he's as committed to fitness and bodybuilding as anyone you'll ever meet in a gym, and he has the physique to prove it. Because bodybuilding emphasizes building muscle and staying lean, Beale was prompted to start experimenting with pyruvate, in part because it's known to facilitate fat loss as well as inhibit weight gain should you happen to overeat. In other words, if you overeat, you'll put on less weight if you're supplementing with pyruvate than if you're not. Beale says,

> It seems we all want to lose weight and have less fat on our bodies—whether we're actually overweight or not. And the fact is that as you get older—I'm now sixty-seven—even if you maintain the same weight as you did when you were twenty, you will have a higher percentage of body fat. And one of the main reasons is the loss of pyruvate from the body as you get older.
>
> Indeed, my waistline did get bigger with age, but I brought it back down—and the only thing I'm doing differently now than I was earlier is I'm weight training consistently and supplementing with pyruvate. Now my waist is smaller than when I was a senior in high school, and it's certainly smaller than when I was playing football at the University of California (Berkeley) in the 1950s.[8]

Heart of the Matter

But as Beale learned through experience, running a lot of miles or lifting a lot of weights as he's done through the years doesn't necessarily safeguard you against health problems. He says:

> My father died of a heart attack at age sixty-one, and I used to be a *horrible* eater of fat. I could just take Kraft Swiss Cheese and eat a whole package. So despite all my years in athletics, I developed a cardiac condition which required five-way multiple bypass surgery in 1991. While my chest pains subsided after the surgery, I never was able to come back to full functionality. I had what they call ischemic (or dead) heart tissue. The only thing I could do was keep taking the medication my doctors gave me and resign myself to the fact that my hardcore athletic days were probably over.
>
> But I had read that pyruvate supplementation could reverse ischemic tissue, which in lay terms is tissue lacking blood supply. So an even more important objective I had in using pyruvate was to see if it would work on my heart.
>
> When I started taking pyruvate, it was more than four years after my surgery and my heart was functioning at only 20 percent. But after about a year of pyruvate supplementation, I went back to my cardiologist and he couldn't believe it! In fact, he gave me extra tests just to make sure his diagnosis was accurate. I didn't have ischemic tissue anymore! In fact, my heart was functioning completely normally at rest, and in exercise tests it was performing so well I was almost off the chart for my age bracket.

So I threw away my heart medication, and I haven't used it since. Now when somebody asks me, "What do you think about pyruvate?" you'd better believe I've got a story to tell them.[9]

Of course, from a purely scientific standpoint, it must be acknowledged that Beale didn't go through a double-blind study in this instance, but the improvement in his heart condition as a result of pyruvate supplementation was more than enough evidence to make a true believer out of him. He's now a manufacturer of calcium pyruvate for the supplement industry and holds several patents on pyruvate formulations. He has also initiated valuable research on pyruvate at his Beale Research Center in San Francisco, California. He says:

> I was semi-retired but the challenge and value of pyruvate brought me out of that fast. If I didn't believe there was tremendous good in pyruvate, I can assure you I wouldn't be using it, not to mention manufacturing and marketing it.
>
> As I said, my story includes the impact pyruvate has had on my heart condition, including the reversal of "dead" or ischemic tissue. It's not uncommon for heart patients to have dead tissue in their heart, and I don't think I need to tell you that ain't good, my friend. But to think that after open heart surgery, when I had what appeared to be per-manent damage, I have completely reversed that perma-nent damage—and there's no other factor that could have been involved other than pyruvate! That is the only thing I changed during that period of time when my heart prob-lems were all but eliminated.[10]

14

2

PYRUVATE: A DEFINITION

Pyruvate, a compound found in our bloodstream and cells at all times, is essential for metabolism. Chemically, pyruvate is composed of carbon, hydrogen and oxygen, which makes it a carbohydrate. Its chemical formula is $CH_3COCOOH$.

A pyruvate molecule contains three carbon atoms and is the breakdown product in the body of the sugar glucose, a six-carbon compound. Essentially, pyruvate is the end product of carbohydrate metabolism in which glucose (a six-carbon molecule) yields two molecules of pyruvate (a three-carbon molecule), or more accurately pyruvic acid. Thus, in the process of human metabolism, pyruvate is the main natural compound which enters the mitochondria, the power plant of the cell, to produce energy.

Pyruvic acid is chemically unstable, so manufacturers stabilize it by adding either calcium, sodium, potassium, magnesium or zinc to form a "salt" called pyruvate. But the manufacture of pyruvate is not simple, which helps explain why the supplement is only now coming on the market.

Perhaps the most amazing thing about pyruvate, research shows, is that if consumed in doses at least two to five times more than the amount normally consumed by the average person, it produces unexpected but highly beneficial metabolic effects. And, of course, since pyruvate is not a drug but a natural compound or metabolite which we consume daily in our diet, pyruvate nutritional supplementation at reasonable dosages should not cause adverse side effects—and this has been verified in human and animal investigations.

Energy Production in the Body

Energy is released from foodstuffs we consume through the process of oxidation. Enzyme systems exist within our body cells which, in a series of steps, convert fats, proteins or carbohydrates into compounds suitable for entering the body's energy-producing cycle. This cycle is the Krebs citric-acid cycle, or Krebs cycle for short (see the following diagram). For example, glycogen is converted into glucose, which in turn is converted to pyruvate, which then enters the mitochondria of the cell. Thus pyruvate is the major compound which produces energy in the mitochondria, sometimes referred to as "the furnace of the body" because it's the energy-producing part of the cell.

When pyruvate is oxidized, the released energy is used to form a high-energy compound called acetylcoenzyme A, which enters the Krebs cycle.

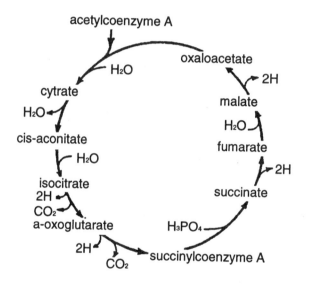

Figure A. THE KREBS CYCLE

The mitochondria of a cell has a system of enzymes. The molecule of "fuel," in this instance acetylcoenzyme A, is handed on from enzyme to enzyme, each enzyme changing it a little bit before passing it on to the next. At most stages, as you can see in the diagram, hydrogen or carbon dioxide is liberated from the molecule.

17

The end result of this cycle is that energy is released along with water. In the body this energy, instead of being lost as heat, is used to link an additional phosphate group to an existing molecule of ADP (adenosine diphosphate) to form the energy-rich compound called ATP (adenosine triphosphate). The ATP is stored and the energy "trapped" in it is used by the body as required. Here are three examples of how that energy is used:

1) To build more complex materials such as protein for use in new tissue growth and repair, and to create secretions and enzymes.
2) For the work of the cell (in ways not fully understood), e.g. muscle contraction and the transmission of nerve impulses.
3) To liberate heat to keep the body warm.

The Krebs citric-acid cycle is the primary pathway by which potential energy stored in food is released by cells in a complex series of chemical reactions to make their own energy-rich compound, ATP. Obviously, pyruvate is a natural and integral part of that process. Who would have expected that supplementing the diet directly with a substance that the body produces naturally would result in such a variety of benefits?

Sources of Pyruvate

Pyruvate is not only found in our bodies at all times, but also occurs naturally in our diet. It is present in abundance in such foods as red apples, cheeses and red wines. Given this information, and the fact that research suggests pyruvate helps prevent disease, one might ask: Does the high pyruvate content of red apples help explain the old saying, "An apple a day keeps the doctor away"?

Furthermore, does the high pyruvate content of red wines and cheeses explain why French people, who are so fond of both, have a lower incidence of heart disease than might be expected? It's food for thought, considering that cheese wouldn't normally fit into the picture of a diet suitable for good cardiac health.

At a recent lecture, noted pyruvate researcher Dr. Ronald Stanko of the University of Pittsburgh said, only partly in jest:

> As a scientist, I'm intrigued by this problem called the "French Paradox." And that is that Frenchmen eat all this fat, they certainly don't exercise as much as we do, and they live longer than we do! What the heck's this all about? I mean, it destroys the fat theory—just totally blows it out of the water! They're eating 43 percent fat a day, we're eating 32 percent fat, and they have less heart disease than we do. So either the United States scientists are completely wrong with this fat theory, which is possible, or the French are doing something that makes them better healthwise.

And what do they do? They drink red wine all day! And they eat cheeses all day! Both of which are high in pyruvate content. My gut feeling is it might have something to do with pyruvate. I really think so.

Right now I'm also trying to figure out where in the heck the idea that eating an apple a day will keep the doctor away came from. Why did anybody ever dream that up? There had to be some basis to that. I mean, some old grandmother must have dreamed that up—why? Were the people who ate apples in the 1600s living longer? I don't know. But again I'd like to find out. You know, what is this all about? Maybe an apple a day will keep the doctor away. Actually, about eight apples a day, right?[11]

Dr. Stanko makes the latter comment because a red apple contains about half a gram of pyruvate and his research indicates that the optimum recommended dosage for pyruvate supplementation is two to five grams daily.[12]

3

The Supporting Research

To protect the American public from manufacturers who produce and sell unsubstantiated dietary products or supplements, Congress passed the Dietary Supplement Act (also known as the "Hatch Act") in 1994. The Hatch Act prohibits the sale of any compound or supplement unless it has been proven to provide a proposed benefit with investigations substantiating those benefits published in what is defined as peer-reviewed literature.

Pyruvate certainly falls into this category. Not only have scientific researchers at the University of Pittsburgh, the United States Armed Forces Medical School, the University of Florida, the University of Texas, Montana State University, Beale Research Center and other institutions studied pyruvate, but the number of papers and studies on pyruvate indexed in scientific and medical information services such as MedLine number in the thousands!

One of the pioneers of pyruvate research in America has been Dr. Stanko, an associate professor of medicine and surgery at the University of Pittsburgh, and a board-certified clinical nutritionist. He started looking at pyruvate in the early 1970s as part of his interest in the control of metabolism and its effect on diseases. Dr. Stanko has described those early beginnings: "I believed in the theory that if we could naturally control what's going on in our body, we might be able to stop some bad things from happening to us. So I took up [the study of pyruvate] in 1972-1973. It's now been twenty-five years that we've been working on this."[13] At the outset Dr. Stanko had eight ideas he wanted to explore regarding metabolism. He explains:

> Seven of them didn't work at all, but one did. And that was an attempt to control our metabolism using high doses or supplementary doses of a compound that's always in your body—that compound, of course, is pyruvate. . . . We know it's the only compound that gets into this energy furnace (the mitochondria). Let's give it in high concentrations and see if we can force the body to do something that it normally does anyway, and make better things happen.
>
> It was a crazy idea at the time. Not accepted by the medical community—that's why it took us twenty-five years to convince them. But it worked! It honest-to-goodness worked. [If] you put this particular product in concentrations of two to five grams a day into your body, what happens is the energy furnace does become more efficient. Now there's a lot of other things that happen afterwards, but that's one thing that we see.[14]

It took Dr. Stanko and his research associates at the University of Pittsburgh about ten years to see that pyruvate supplementation does indeed "make the body's energy furnace more efficient," as he puts it. As it turns out, a physiologist named Rolf Bunger, a German citizen who works at the United States Armed Forces Medical School in Bethesda, Maryland, was doing essentially the same research at the same time—and getting the same results! Dr. Stanko says:

> I didn't know he was doing the same work. I was working in Pittsburgh, he was working in Washington, D.C. Oh, we met each other every once in a while, but we wouldn't tell each other anything.
>
> It was an inefficient way to do research, but what it did was twenty years later, when we both got old, here were these two scientists who had both found the same thing. And in the scientific community—that means the old, established medical community that we are both a part of—unless more than one guy does it, nobody believes it. I mean, I might be the nicest guy in the world, but nobody will believe just one scientist—no matter what data he has!
>
> So Bunger was doing his work—he's a good scientist, and he's got great data—and I was doing mine. And we found the same thing: this stuff [pyruvate] does increase cellular energy when you take it.[15]

4

BENEFITS OF
PYRUVATE

In the years that have passed since Dr. Stanko and Dr. Bunger did their early studies, they and numerous other researchers at different institutions have continued the research on pyruvate and uncovered a veritable cornucopia of benefits. So many, in fact, one could say that pyruvate's cup runneth over with value previously unforeseen. The following is a list of some of the key benefits attributed to its usage (many of them supported by patents):

• Enhanced exercise capacity or endurance
• Increased energy in the muscle cell
• Enhanced fat loss
• Enhanced weight loss (*Note:* Weight loss is not necessarily fat loss, since you can actually lose weight and increase your percentage of body fat.)
• Decreased weight gain when overeating

- Increased lean body mass
- Inhibition of ischemic heart and intestinal injury
- Decreased heart tissue damage after heart attack
- Decreased osteoporosis
- Increased heart efficiency, so the heart is able to pump blood without needing, or using, as much oxygen
- Decreased perception of workload
- Enhanced efficiency of electrolyte and thirst-quenching drinks
- Enhanced effectiveness of protein powder
- Decreased blood glucose in diabetics
- Decrease in eye disease among diabetics
- Lower-than-expected cholesterol levels when consuming a high-fat diet
- Inhibited production of free radicals, which have been identified as damaging agents in many diseases and the aging process
- Scavenging of free radicals already in the body
- Inhibition of cancerous tumors
- Prevention of cellular destruction
- Decreased muscle degradation in AIDS and other forms of catabolic disease
- In solution, pyruvate stabilizes organs for long periods of time for use in transplantation and inhibits rejection of transplanted organs

Each manufacturer of pyruvate-based products, whether the product is in capsule, powder or drink form, inevitably includes different additives to help facilitate specific benefits or to simply differentiate their product from others on the market. The above list of benefits is not available collectively in any one pyruvate-based product.

This publication is intended to introduce the overall or generic benefits of pyruvate. No one manufacturer of pyruvate will create a pyruvate product targeted at meeting all the beneficial claims of pyruvate, either due to restrictions imposed by patents, patents pending, or by choice. Read the label on your purchased product to determine the product's purpose. A few of the above listed claims involve prescriptions, and those that don't are not intended to diagnose, treat or cure any disease.

5

UNANSWERED QUESTIONS

Despite all the benefits attributed to pyruvate, several unanswered questions exist regarding the supplement and its effects:

- Will pyruvate taken in small doses produce weight loss as advertised? The published studies on pyruvate which show enhanced weight loss had the subjects taking very high dosages—twenty-six grams a day. No one has proved to date that pyruvate will produce the same weight loss at much smaller dosages such as two to five grams, yet that's what the advertising implies.

- Does pyruvate work by itself, or only in combination with other substances? In many published studies, subjects were given pyruvate in combination with other substances—dihydroxyacetone (DHA), for example.

Thus it may not be technically correct to infer from such studies that pyruvate alone produced the benefits demonstrated. Of course, there are many substances that don't work by themselves, but they work synergistically. No one seems to dispute the fact that pyruvate plus other substances produces benefits, but there is some debate on how effective pyruvate is on its own.

• If pyruvate is so effective as a weight-loss supplement, why are there only two studies—one on a sedentary group of overweight women taking twenty-six grams a day, and another on a group of rats—which demonstrate a weight loss? The skeptical point of view is that if the supplement works so effectively to enhance weight loss, there should be numerous studies proving it. In fact, that is not the case, and the absence of such studies over time is troubling.

• What relevance does animal research concerning pyruvate have for humans? Many experts agree that it is very difficult to apply data from animal studies to humans, though many also agree that it is difficult to conduct initial research with human subjects. The fact that a substantial portion of the pyruvate research has been done on animals only adds to the question marks regarding pyruvate's effectiveness.

• Finally, why did the giant pharmaceutical company, Abbott-Ross Laboratories, lose interest in pyruvate after spending millions of dollars on research? A possible explanation may be that their studies didn't support the claims, or at least didn't support them to their satisfaction.

The important thing to realize is that whether or not the research on pyruvate has categorically proven the benefits attributed to the supplement, it is suggested that people consider trying pyruvate experimentally to ascertain if it works for them. After all, since pyruvate is a nontoxic, natural substance, there should be no downside, other than the expense factor, in trying the supplement. And in view of the many benefits attributed to pyruvate, such experimentation may be well worth it.

6

FASTER, HIGHER, STRONGER

The 1996 Atlanta Olympic Games are still fresh on all our minds, and the motto of the Olympics is— *Faster, Higher, Stronger.* How many athletes, whether they're Olympians, would-be Olympians or simply "weekend warriors," wouldn't perk up and take notice upon hearing Dr. Stanko's comment that "this stuff does increase cellular energy when you take it"? It is not surprising that pyruvate is expected to become one of the most popular supplements in sports nutrition.

The pursuit of excellence in athletics, whether we're talking about the Olympics or merely a 10K race in the neighborhood, is, in large measure, the creation of increased energy and endurance through conscientious training, good nutrition, proper rest, etc. Clinical studies at the University of Pittsburgh School of Medicine and Abbott-Ross Laboratories have shown that pyruvate supplementation increased endurance levels by up to 20 percent—a startling improvement and one which is particularly great news to athletes in sports where endurance is a factor.[16]

These studies have shown, through muscle biopsies and blood samples, that pyruvate dramatically increases energy and endurance capacity by facilitating greater glucose utilization. When the supply of blood glucose is depleted, the body will utilize intra-muscular glucose.

This enhanced utilization of glucose delays the onset of fatigue, which will obviously help athletes perform better in competition. But that is not all. By extending one's submaximal endurance capacity (it has also been reported that pyruvate supplementation results in higher concentrations of glycogen being stored in the liver and in muscle), pyruvate allows an athlete to train longer and at a higher intensity. Since training ultimately makes the athlete, pyruvate gives athletes a double advantage—enhanced performance in competition, and more effective training in preparation for competition.

Pyruvate offers some other exciting benefits to athletes. Studies conducted by Dr. Robert Cade and his associates at the University of Florida show that pyruvate supplementation reduces perceived workload in athletics—or in any kind of physical task for that matter. Whether you're doing a hard running workout on a track or challenging yourself with weights in a gym, the effort seems to be easier if you have been supplementing with pyruvate. Perhaps that's to be expected since pyruvate increases the energy capacity of muscle cells. Nonetheless, it's no mean benefit considering how important the psychological factor is in athletics.

Perhaps related to the lower perceived workload, pyruvate also seems to be a modest mood elevator, i.e., you feel better psychologically as well as physically. Greater energy and endurance, lower perceived workload, a slight mood elevator—clearly there's more than enough here to make the athlete take a hard look at pyruvate as a nutritional supplement. What athlete in his right mind wouldn't?

Pax Beale emphasizes the positives of pyruvate as follows: "Since it is an innocuous supplement, being a naturally occurring product in the body—it doesn't affect the central nervous system, doesn't make you break out in sweat, doesn't give you acne or pimples, and doesn't make your heart race—it's the type of substance that athletes and others can use and deploy to their benefit in an infinite number of ways.

The Body Beautiful

The increased energy and endurance pyruvate offers is obviously of great benefit in athletic performance. But the enhanced weight loss it also produces, as well as some other benefits pertaining to lean muscle mass, make it equally attractive in another way. Call it aesthetics or, if you will, building the body beautiful.

"Pyruvate has a definite impact on how we look cosmetically," says Pax Beale, "that is, lean body mass. The body itself, when it gets toned (i.e., as you increase muscle and decrease fat), that's called a lean body mass and that makes a more aesthetic body. So muscle, or a toned body, is aesthetically attractive, and fat isn't. And we are forever fighting that issue."[17]

Given Beale's involvement with bodybuilding, it should come as no surprise that he and his associates at the Beale Research Center in San Francisco have experimented extensively on combining pyruvate with other substances in an effort to create pyruvate-based supplements particularly suitable for that sport. Not that pyruvate alone isn't an appropriate nutritional supplement for bodybuilders, but Beale's thinking goes beyond the simplistic concept of taking some capsules of pyruvate or anything else to lose a few pounds. He thinks in terms of synergy, the combined action of things, and anyone who really understands the process of achieving weight loss, all-round health and having an aesthetic, attractive body knows intuitively he's probably on the right track. Says Beale:

> Pyruvate alone can help you lose weight if you take it in sufficient quantities, but as I've often said before, God has not given you a pill that you can't out-eat if you want to. Therefore, the best way to approach the challenge of losing weight and having a toned, aesthetic, muscular body is to use a combination of exercise, nutrition and pyruvate supplementation—perhaps with other substances added to pyruvate for synergistic effect.

What we have found is that if you combine pyruvate with what they call an anticortisol/anticatabolic agent such as DHEA, phosphatidylserine (PS) or a number of others we have experimented with, you get the best of both worlds—a supplement that helps you burn fat and build muscle at the same time.[18]

He explains that when you work out intensely by lifting weights, you, in fact, damage the muscles. The *catabolic* phase is when muscles break down. The *anabolic* phase is when muscle is mended or rebuilt. Beale asks:

Why not put something in [the pyruvate supplement] that decreases the muscle breakdown from intense training—in other words, an anticatabolic agent? If you're able to train just as hard and you don't have the amount of muscle damage that you otherwise would, you start at a higher plateau in the anabolic process taking place between your workouts where the real muscle growth or gain occurs.

Just a side comment: Anabolic steroids, everybody knows, build muscle when used in combination with intense weight training. (Please understand I'm not advocating the use of steroids here; I'm just illustrating a point.) Then along comes a product like human growth hormone (HGH), which laboratory-wise is considerably more anabolic that most anabolic steroids. Yet anabolic steroids produce more muscle than HGH does, and nobody could figure out why.

Then they found that inherent in certain anabolic steroids that were good for muscle building was an anticatabolic component. That is, it prevented the muscle from breaking down as much during the workout. So the net effect of combining that anti-catabolic effect with the anabolic nature of steroids yielded better results than HGH, which was more anabolic but didn't have an anti-catabolic component.[19]

Beale and his associates have been experimenting with combining pyruvate with the aforementioned anti-catabolic agents to produce a product specifically geared for serious bodybuilders and other athletes involved in anaerobic sports such as sprinting, weightlifting, throwing the shot putt or discus, etc. He feels that for athletes who are involved in less intense or aerobic activity, this combination of ingredients in a supplement probably won't be particularly effective because the anti-catabolic characteristics are primarily suited for intense, anaerobic exercise. In other words, an aerobic-oriented person or someone interested in moderate fitness probably wouldn't gain maximum benefit from it. Clearly, what Beale and his team are researching is a specialty product for hardcore bodybuilders. He adds:

> We've also done some research on combining pyruvate with hydroxycitric acid (HCA), found in the herb *Garcinia cambogia*, and we feel this also has tremendous potential. This product would be suitable to anyone, regardless of the type of exercise the person does.
>
> In studies on rats, *Garcinia cambogia* works as an appetite suppressant. In all candor, so I'm not taken out of context, the garcinia tests on humans are anecdotal, although the tests are very supportive in animals. Therefore, you're not going to find me going out on a limb

saying unequivocally that there are double-blind studies and you can take it to the bank that the combination of pyruvate and HCA has a synergistic effect that makes each one of them, together, work better than either one would alone. But there's enough evidence to lean in that direction. And, of course, pyruvate can work by itself—in high enough dosages. But if you combine it with HCA, it is our theory that you don't have to take as much pyruvate supplementation as you otherwise would.[20]

Obviously, the main thrust of Beale's approach has been an attempt to combine different ingredients synergistically to create more effective pyruvate-based supplements—maybe even create what could be called designer supplements with pyruvate as the main ingredient. He states:

> . . . Clearly, when you combine pyruvate with other products such as phosphatidylserine or HCA and there are a host of others out there, such as CLA (conjugated linoleic acid) and the amino acid leucine, you can get an interesting synergistic effect. When you then use these pyruvate-based supplements in conjunction with exercise and proper nutrition, it's like bringing all these things together. And I don't think there's any doubt about it—you've got yourself an optimum weight control-fat loss-increased lean body mass program.
>
> The exercise is necessary because no matter how good your nutrition or how much pyruvate supplementation you take, you're not going to gain muscle or have a toned body unless you do some exercise. And muscle shapes the body positively, fat doesn't. So it's not a question of just losing weight. In fact, you can lose weight and gain fat! How? By burning or losing muscle. It's not even a question of just losing fat.

What you want to do is lose fat and gain muscle, and make the ratio between muscle and fat wider. The greater the difference between muscle mass and fat, the more aesthetic your body. That's just a fact of life.

And a factor of getting there is nutrition . . . basically a diet low in fat and relatively high in protein and complex carbohydrates is best. But you bring all these things together as I said, and they have a dynamic, synergistic effect.[21]

Pyruvate and Electrolyte Replacement

At the University of Florida Dr. Robert Cade and his associates have done extensive research on how pyruvate could be used to enhance the value and effectiveness of electrolyte replacement drinks such as Gatorade, which Dr. Cade invented. The results of that research are so positive that Dr. Cade and his team now have five patents on pyruvate—all related to improving the quality of electrolyte drinks. Essentially their research shows that an electrolyte-pyruvate mixture is better than an electrolyte drink alone in the recovery process during exercise.[22]

Electrolytes are various minerals in the body—primarily potassium, phosphorus, magnesium, zinc and sodium—crucial to proper physiological function. When you perspire, you not only lose water, you also lose electrolytes. If you perspire very heavily and lose too many electrolytes, you become weak. In rare and extreme cases, you could even die.

For athletes or anyone who exercises strenuously it's very important to maintain electrolyte balance—particularly if you're doing something over a prolonged period of time, such as running a marathon, playing football, basketball, soccer or tennis on a hot day, etc.

Electrolyte drinks (and there are many of them, Gatorade being the best known) are obviously superior to straight water in facilitating the recovery of individuals who have experienced electrolyte loss. The research done by Dr. Cade and his associates indicates that when pyruvate is added to the electrolyte drink, it enhances that recovery even more—and the improvement is dramatic. Unfortunately, despite the patents that clearly show pyruvate would be an extremely beneficial additive to electrolyte drinks, there are no pyruvate-enhanced drinks on the market to date.

7

A Dieter's Dream?

A lot of excitement has been generated over pyruvate as a "weight loss breakthrough." This type of language leads people to assume that maybe this—finally!—is that long-awaited magic pill which will give them the lean body they want. One ad that has appeared in a Los Angeles area newspaper proclaims:[23]

FORGET PHEN-FEN & LOSE WEIGHT NOW WITH PYRUVATE

New BREAKTHROUGH Weight Loss Product, Safe, effective alternative to Phen-Fen

PYRUVATE	PHEN-FEN/REDUX
1. Naturally Reoccurring Nutrient	1. Class 4 Drug
2. No Side Effects	2. Dangerous Side Effects
3. No Prescription Needed	3. Prescription Required
4. Potent Antioxidant	4. No Benefit
5. Protects Lean Muscle	5. No Benefit
6. Increases Endurance	6. No Benefit

On the face of it, absolutely nothing this ad says is inaccurate. However, there is an all-important gray area between "fact" and "promised benefits" where it's possible for a person to get lost or jump to the wrong conclusion.

Dr. Stanko explains the possible mechanism by which pyruvate supplementation burns fat and and causes weight loss (and reduced weight gain should you overeat):

> Pyruvate in higher concentrations is getting into what is called the citric-acid cycle, or Krebs cycle, and you burn fat—as you're making the energy, you burn fat. What we have found in human studies, and in some animal studies, is that along with that, you don't synthesize as much fat. So the end point of supplementing with pyruvate is that you do have more ATP or energy, but also we found that you don't maintain as much body fat, which is nice, because everybody wants to be thinner.[24]

Indeed, studies have shown that pyruvate supplementation significantly enhances weight and fat loss while on a low-calorie diet. A study at the University of Pittsburgh and Montefiore University on fourteen overweight women supplementing their diet with a high daily dosage of pyruvate produced these results: "Subjects fed pyruvate showed a greater weight and fat loss than the group fed simply a low-energy diet. The group receiving pyruvate demonstrated an average of 37 percent greater weight loss and 48 percent greater fat loss compared to the placebo group."[25]

Of course, the hidden problem with any weight-reduction program is keeping the weight off once you've lost it.

That, countless dieters will tell you, is the hard part! Since pyruvate has also been shown to inhibit weight and fat gain with resumption of higher calorie eating after losing the original weight, it seems to be the ideal supplement for both losing the weight and keeping it off—in other words, a dieter's dream.

There is some sobering information a dieter should know, however. As previously mentioned, the tests showing that pyruvate enhances weight and fat loss were done at very high dosages—twenty-six grams a day. So it can be said we know pyruvate works to enhance weight loss, but at what dosage? Or as one cynic has put it, "Of course, you'll lose weight by taking twenty-six grams of pyruvate a day! Your stomach will be so upset, you won't be able to eat anything."

Secondly, even if an individual, through experimentation, finds a more moderate dosage that works effectively for weight loss and weight control, it should be noted that pyruvate, at best, simply enhances the process of weight loss. It makes sense that it works best if the individual also exercises consistently. It is not, in and of itself, a magic shortcut.

Furthermore, referring back to the study mentioned above, it's important to note that the women were already on a restricted diet which was producing a weight loss. The pyruvate supplementation simply augmented that weight loss. Remember that 48 percent fat loss? This means that if a person on a diet or weight-loss program lost two pounds of fat without pyruvate, the weight loss would have been three pounds with pyruvate supplementation. Significant, but not necessarily meaningful if the person taking pyruvate isn't on a diet or a weight-loss program causing a reduction of weight in the first place. Because—do the math—what is a 48 percent greater weight loss than zero (which would be the weight loss if a person wasn't in a weight-loss mode already)? The answer, of course, is zero!

The point is that pyruvate, at least based on this study, should be viewed as a weight loss accelerator when you've already put the pieces of the formula into place to start losing weight in the first place, whether it's an increase in exercise, a reduction in caloric intake, etc. Not that it isn't a big advantage, of course, to be able to take a nutritional supplement which will accelerate a weight loss already in progress.

However, it must be reported that thus far pyruvate has not been shown to produce significant weight loss if you supplement your diet with it and merrily go on your way consuming a high-fat, high-calorie diet and living a totally sedentary lifestyle. You may want to believe that pyruvate all by itself (shades of that magic pill idea) will take care of the problem through some miracle of physiology. But it won't happen; at least there's nothing in any studies conducted thus far which says it will.

This brings us to a claim made by the executive of a company which markets pyruvate that he lost thirty-nine pounds in forty days by taking the supplement and doing nothing else—no reduction in caloric intake, no increase in exercise, nothing! Such a claim, by any standard of logic or physiology, strains the bounds of believability to say the least.

Pax Beale, who has an extensive knowledge of nutrition, weight loss and weight control as befits someone who's been a champion bodybuilder, doesn't mince words in assessing this individual's claim:

> I consider it a complete fraud. This man was actually quoted as saying that he lost thirty-nine pounds in forty days without changing his nonexercise lifestyle and while continuing to eat the same good-quality, oily foods that he ate before! Well, rumor has it this individual tips the scales at 300 pounds, so that probably means it would be easier for him to lose more weight faster than somebody who weighed 100 pounds.
>
> Notwithstanding that, my own personal opinion is that if you had this guy take a lie detector test, you'd see he was lying. He's made that claim because he wants to sell his company's product. But the odds of a person losing thirty-nine pounds of fat in forty days—I'm not talking about water loss or anything like that; you couldn't lose thirty-nine pounds of water and live—are so remote it's just plain unbelievable. Think of it, losing thirty-nine pounds in forty days—that's almost a pound a day—without so much as touching your diet or exercise level; there's no way that could happen.
>
> And why am I even taking the time to discuss this man's ridiculous claim? Because I know pyruvate is a good product. You don't have to go out and be a con artist and try to sell it with malarkey like that.[26]

So the picture seems clear. First, if you're on a decreased calorie diet and you supplement with pyruvate, you'll lose more weight than you would otherwise. But that doesn't necessarily mean you'll lose a lot of weight simply using pyruvate without decreasing your caloric intake or increasing your exercise level.

Second, if you overeat while supplementing with pyruvate, you'll gain less weight than you would otherwise—but it doesn't mean you won't gain any weight.

Third, pyruvate won't produce a significant weight loss by itself; you have to help it along. What that means is that if you want to use pyruvate to lose weight, the recommended approach is to reduce your caloric intake (not necessarily by eating less food, but eating more high-fiber, low-calorie foods), increase your exercise level (not only to burn calories, but also speed up your metabolism), and supplement with pyruvate to accelerate the whole process. That combination can and will produce dramatic results.

As Pax Beale puts it, "When somebody comes up to me and asks, 'What's the ideal weight-loss program?' I say, 'It's nutrition, it's exercise, and tweaking the process with pyruvate.' That's utopia!" Pyruvate is apparently a nice supplement to "tweak the process" of losing fat or keeping your weight under control, but you can out-eat it. You will get fat, whether you're supplementing with pyruvate or not, if you just start eating butter, mayonnaise and every other fatty food you can get your hands on, while living the life of a couch potato.

8

FREE RADICALS, DISEASE & AGING

As all of us know, considerable attention has been focused in recent years on the negative health effects of free radicals, those unstable, reactive substances that can cause severe damage to cell structure. Free radicals, which attack cell walls and reduce the cell's ability to function and regulate itself, have been implicated in a vast variety of diseases and health conditions ranging from arthritis and malignancy to general aging.

At one time it appeared that antioxidants such as vitamin A, vitamin C, vitamin E and various minerals held great promise in combatting free radicals, but now it appears in some situations they're only marginally effective.

Pyruvate, however, has been proven in studies on mammals to be both a free radical scavenger and inhibitor. It is effective in both destroying these sinister substances and, even more importantly, preventing their production in the first place. The latter should be emphasized because there are various substances that supposedly act as free radical scavengers in the body, but pyruvate is the first substance. that apparently acts as a free radical inhibitor.

Talking about the history of the research on free radicals, Dr. Stanko says:

> When I went to medical school, we never heard of free radicals. Then the first free radical study came from Czechoslovakia about fifteen or eighteen years ago. It was just a one-page article, sort of like the article announcing the discovery of DNA. But nobody believed it, because the study came from Czechoslovakia. But the American scientific community then took up on it, and they found [a free radical] is a real entity. The top scientists in the world now are convinced that free radicals are not good for you.[27]

Considering how often we hear about free radicals, it's curious that so few of us have any idea what they are. Exactly what is a free radical?

We breathe oxygen (O_2), which combines with pyruvate (CCC, a three-carbon molecule) in the mitochondria to create energy (ATP) so we can stay alive. "That's why we breathe," explains Dr. Stanko. "I mean, you breathe for one reason only—to feed that mitochondria to make the ATP. When you don't have any oxygen, you can't do it."

Normally the body is about 97 percent efficient in using up the oxygen we breathe, but that leaves 3 percent unaccounted for, and therein lies the problem. In a recent lecture he gave to the Sterling Health Group in Dallas, Dr. Stanko illustrated what happens:

> This [O_2] is stable, it doesn't hurt you. It actually keeps you alive. But a free radical would be [O_1]. This is an oxygen molecule with a free electron, and is a very unstable product. It's not good to have around. [O_2] keeps you alive, it [O_1] goes around and breaks down a lot of things (i.e., O_1).
>
> Free radicals have now been associated with almost every disease you can imagine. Initially, when you see something like that—just like when you see the beneficial effects of pyruvate—you say, "Hey, this can't be true!" I mean, not *everything* is related to free radicals. But in reality it looks like a lot of the bad things that happen to us are related to that.
>
> Rheumatoid arthritis—there's a lot of evidence that free radicals are what causes the breakdown of the joints in rheumatoid arthritis. There's no question that ischemic heart disease, which all of us now really fear—that's the number one disease in our country, along with malignancy—is related to an overabundance of free radicals. And malignancy is related to free radicals.[28]

Since free radicals are a fact of life, a by-product of breathing, the very act that keeps us alive, what is to be done about them? The good news is that the body has some important allies to combat these unstable, destructive molecules. We know these allies are, of course, antioxidants, which we take in through our diet as well as through supplementation. The bad news is that antioxidants don't seem to be working very effectively. Dr. Stanko explains:

Normally the body has 97 percent of [O_2] and 3 percent of [O_1], and we have in our body what we call antioxidants, which you've heard a zillion things about—vitamin C, vitamin A, all kinds of them. In actuality, probably the one that is working best as an antioxidant is vitamin E. That's the one that's been shown to be effective in some very large studies.

What these antioxidants do is get rid of [O_1]—the free radical. They come in, attack this free radical, and take it away. But the question comes up: All right, everybody's taking antioxidants, why are they not working? Vitamin E is the only one right now that seems to be very, very good. But why don't they always work?

Well, what happens is that [O_1] is so active that even when you take an antioxidant, the antioxidants can be beneficial but the free radicals are still doing damage. You have to prevent the free radical from being made in the first place. And there has been no way to prevent free radicals from happening because it's a normal thing that goes on in your body at all times.[29]

Nothing to prevent free radicals from being formed until now—or so it appears. Dr. Stanko continues:

One thing that we found is that when you take pyruvate, in high concentrations again, what happens is that for whatever reason—and we are not sure why this happens—but we now know for sure your body doesn't make free radicals. See, that's the key. You don't have that bad thing (O_1) running around, so then the antioxidant has to come and take it away. It's not there to begin with.[30]

The ramifications of this boggle the mind, considering the havoc free radicals supposedly wreak in our bodies. The Nobel Prize was seemingly designed for scientific discoveries like this! Yet despite these research findings regarding pyruvate and free radicals, Dr. Stanko stops short of claiming this as a benefit of the substance, at least for now. He says:

> The thing about pyruvate we have held back for a long, long, long, long time is that it was just sounding too good—and if you want to really anger the medical community, come out and make promises. They'll jump all over you. I would, too. That's what I do for a living, all right? I review [the literature and findings] and if it doesn't sound for real, I say, "Hey, I'm not going to accept it."
>
> So we have repeated this research over and over and over again. And it's for real, it happens. So we do have evidence now, in animals, in many animal studies, that we can inhibit free radicals from being made.[31]

Slowing the Aging Process

If indeed pyruvate can prevent free radical formation in the body, this not only means it could be a strong line of defense against disease, but perhaps a way to slow the aging process itself. Says Dr. Stanko:

You've probably heard the theory that aging is secondary to free radicals. And what is that theory based on? Well, [O₁] again, floating around for fifty years in your body, probably does something bad to your DNA, does something bad to your collagen. One of the things that happens to you when you age and your face gets looking wrinkled is that the collagen is changing. And some people feel it's related to free radicals.

So we looked at aging cells. These studies are going on right now along with the cancer studies and transplant studies we're doing. The studies are not completed. But in studying facial cells, these cells get worse if you bombard them with free radicals, they get better if you take the free radicals away, and they really don't get bad at all if you inhibit these free radicals from developing by putting some pyruvate in.

Now these are very preliminary studies, we haven't published anything about it yet. And we're not claiming that pyruvate will stop or slow down aging.[32]

All of us, of course, are free to hope for the best. Could pyruvate supplementation, in fact, be a nutritional fountain of youth? Could it be a much needed measure of prevention against disease? Only time and more research will tell.

9

CANCER
PREVENTION

Studies at the University of Pittsburgh in which malignant tumors were implanted in rats showed that tumor growth was slowed in the animals on pyruvate supplementation versus a placebo group.[33] The reason for this, ostensibly, was pyruvate's effectiveness as a free radical fighter.

The researchers hypothesized that pyruvate inhibits malignant growth by functioning as a free radical inhibitor and scavenger. In this way it might inhibit tumor growth by reducing DNA injury resulting from oxidative stress. Data from these studies indicates that DNA breaks (damage to the genetic material) were reduced 40 percent by pyruvate.

Dr. Ronald Stanko told the Sterling Health Group in Dallas:

Everybody's afraid of cancer or malignancy, and there's a theory that because we are bombarded all our life with that bad free radical (O_1), that's one way you get cancer—that after twenty-seven years of that bad thing running around, it does something bad to you and you get a tumor.

So maybe that free radical, if we can prevent it from happening by using pyruvate, could have some effect on malignancy. If I took a tumor, stuck it on an animal, then fed the animal pyruvate to prevent free radicals from happening, if the theory is correct that tumor should grow less or it should go away. Either one.

Well, we did that. We took a rat (because you have to work on animals in cancer research, you can't work with humans) and had a breast tumor stuck on the rat. We fed him pyruvate, and we looked at free radicals. And we fed him other antioxidants that will take away existing free radicals—besides inhibiting free radicals, we also wanted to take them away.

And what we found, over a period of about ten days, is that when we didn't give the rat pyruvate, the tumor grew rapidly. But when we fed him pyruvate, it grew much slower. Now it didn't go away, but it was one-third the size.

So that was very interesting. Is this going to mean anything [in the fight against cancer]? I'm not sure. I can just tell you that tumors don't grow as well when there's pyruvate around. So that may be of some benefit someday, but the important thing is—it goes back to the free radical theory—inhibition of free radicals is probably good for you.[34]

Of course, an important piece in the complicated puzzle that cancer represents is DNA. Whether it relates to the free radicals or not, DNA is considered to be a key factor in malignancy. Dr. Stanko explains:

We've repeated that study again, and actually looked at the DNA. DNA is genetic material. We looked at rats' genetic material after one week with a tumor growing on them. In the control group of animals (that weren't on pyruvate), the DNA was all broken up and bad—and that's the theory behind cancer, that you get bad DNA which tells your body to do bad things to itself, probably secondary to the free radicals. But the rats that were fed pyruvate had normal looking DNA, which is really something!

Again, I have no idea what this means, but it's good, right? I don't know what's going to happen to you down the line with it, because good DNA is probably the best thing that can happen to you, but am I going to say it's going to make you feel better or prevent cancer—I don't know. But it's a nice finding.[35]

As Dr. Stanko himself would admit, these studies do not even begin to address the question whether pyruvate supplementation might actually prevent tumors in the first place—as one might reasonably expect considering that free radicals have been implicated as a cause of cancer

Obviously, more detailed and long-range studies need to be done in this area, but at this point pyruvate supplementation would seem to be a worthwhile preventive approach where cancer and other diseases are concerned. This is especially the case since, again, pyruvate is a natural substance with no adverse side-effects when taken in sensible dosages.

10

PYRUVATE, DIABETES AND CHOLESTEROL

Diabetes is a major health problem in the United States and is characterized by excessive blood sugar levels. Diabetics are required to take insulin to counteract those elevated levels. Research has shown that pyruvate supplementation for diabetics results in significantly lower glucose values in glucose tolerance tests commonly used to test for diabetes.

In a typical glucose tolerance test an individual is given seventy-five grams of pure glucose orally. The subject's blood glucose is measured right afterwards and then at intervals for the next three hours. Blood glucose values above 200 or thereabouts after sixty minutes indicates probability of a diabetic condition.

When a glucose tolerance test was administered at the University of Pittsburgh Medical School to one diabetic after the individual had supplemented his diet for seven days with 52 grams per day of pyruvate and dihydroxyacetone (DHA) in equal parts, orally administered, the results were as follows:[36]

GLUCOSE TOLERANCE TEST

Time (Minutes)	Blood Glucose without Pyruvate	Blood Glucose with Pyruvate Supplementation
0	104	96
30	155	134
60	213	193
120	245	237
180	204	183

Will pyruvate supplementation prevent diabetes? That's not a question anyone can answer right now. We do know, however, that pyruvate supplementation as ongoing therapy can decrease blood glucose in diabetic patients, and blood cholesterol in individuals with hyperlipidimia. This, in itself, is promising news.

Effect on Cholesterol and Coronary Disease

Research has shown that pyruvate supplementation of a high-fat, high-cholesterol diet will decrease LDL cholesterol (the so-called "bad" cholesterol) in the blood without affecting the HDL ("good") cholesterol concentration.[37] The implications regarding heart attacks and associated coronary problems are obvious, since plasma lipid concentrations are a known risk factor in atherosclerotic heart disease.

Pyruvate seems to have little effect on plasma lipids in normal-weight people consuming a low-cholesterol, low-fat diet, but people who fall into this category are less likely to suffer heart attacks and other coronary problems in the first place.

Another result of pyruvate supplementation, studies show, is a decrease in resting heart rate and diastolic blood pressure. This is a predictable result considering that pyruvate has been shown to improve muscle endurance—and the heart, after all, is a muscle. So one of the benefits of pyruvate supplementation is that cardiac output (the amount of blood pumped by the heart per minute) is increased by increasing stroke volume (amount of blood pumped by the heart each time it contracts). This reduces the oxygen requirement of the heart, allowing it to perform its normal functions more easily.

Clearly, this is an advantage to people involved in athletics as well as to those in the general population who want to enjoy greater cardiac efficiency and protection against coronary problems.

11

CARDIAC ISCHEMIA

Pyruvate has been shown to inhibit ischemic injury and, as Pax Beale's experience demonstrates so dramatically, it facilitates recuperation and repair following such injury. In addition, pyruvate's positive effects on cardiac function also make it a valuable form of therapy in the event of cardiac crisis.[38]

In the case of heart surgery, a liquid drip pyruvate solution (two to twenty grams pyruvate per liter of solution) may be administered during surgery and afterwards until the patient is stabilized. Of course, when time is available, a patient would be wise to take oral dosages of pyruvate for days or weeks prior to anticipated cardiac surgery. Just prior to, during, and after the surgery the liquid drip pyruvate solution could be administered.

Finally, people experiencing congestive heart failure are urged to take regular oral dosages of pyruvate to decrease heart rate, increase stroke volume and reduce oxygen demands of the heart.

No less than 50 percent of the deaths in this country are attributed to heart attack and other coronary problems. Think of it! Every second person you know is going to die of heart problems. Given the severity of the situation, pyruvate is more than worthy of serious consideration as a nutritional supplement.

In animal studies conducted by Dr. Stanko and his research team, animals were given pyruvate supplementation and heart attacks were then induced by clamping off specific blood vessels. The results were notable—there was no ischemic tissue damage. Apparently, in addition to decreasing tissue damage resulting from heart attack, pyruvate also inhibits ischemic heart disease. Dr. Stanko says:

> When we feed [the rats] pyruvate, they don't get the damage. I mean, they really don't. We showed this in three studies. Again, if you look at the old, old medical literature, the 1930s and 1940s, somebody had done a study in Italy in like 1935 hypothesizing this would happen, but they did such a terrible study it never was accepted. But they found very similar data to what we found: that if you stop this free radical from being made by supplementing with pyruvate, you can inhibit ischemic heart disease.[39]

As a final step in a kind of cardiac triple play of benefits, pyruvate has also been shown to produce dramatic results when used in organ transplantation. Dr. Stanko, who has had first-hand experience in this area since he's now work-

ing in the organ transplantation division at the University
of Pittsburgh Medical Center, explains:

> The ultimate ischemic organ is the transplanted organ.
> If you take a person's liver out, put it over here, and then
> transplant it into another person, there's no oxygen going
> to the organ when it's outside the body, so it's completely
> ischemic. And by the time it's transplanted into the new
> person, it's even more ischemic. So that's the ultimate
> organ that's deficient in oxygen.
>
> But if you bathe that organ with pyruvate, or if you
> were to feed the person pyruvate prior to taking the organ
> out, or if you feed the other person pyruvate prior to trans-
> planting the organ into him, the organ's better off. It's
> unbelievable! When you do this, it works. It's unbelievable,
> this ischemic heart idea. It works with your liver and other
> organs the same way.[40]

Based on the research, there seems little doubt that regular pyruvate supplementation is an advisable preventive
measure against heart attack and other coronary problems.
After all, any supplement which is beneficial in controlling
plasma lipid concentrations among people who can't
adhere to a low-cholesterol diet has got to be a major
advantage. Not to mention that—as indicated earlier—
pyruvate supplementation has also been shown to increase
weight loss, as well as inhibit weight gain from overeating.
Indeed, one might ask: What better supplement could
people take to lower their coronary risks?

12

THE SAFETY OF PYRUVATE

No clinical, toxological or marketing studies have shown any serious side effects from pyruvate usage.[18] Diarrhea and gurgling stomach noises were a side effect of pyruvate supplementation with a significant number of people in the early high-dose studies of twenty-six grams a day or more, but the problem has been greatly reduced as lower dosages have become the norm and the quality of pyruvate that is manufactured has improved tremendously.

However, as a precaution, until further studies have been done, pyruvate supplements are not recommended for pregnant women. And as is the case with any supplement taken in pharmacological doses, a physician should be consulted before embarking on a major supplementation program.

Even with the improvements in the quality of pyruvate on the market, it is reported that at dosages of eighteen to twenty grams or more a day, people may experience slight nausea and stomach gas. If you're using higher dosages of pyruvate and that happens, simply lower the dosage temporarily until the problem disappears, and then creep back up in dosage so your body adapts.

It's also important to mention that while pyruvate has been extensively researched and there seem to be no adverse side effects other than the gastrointestinal problems noted, there is really no effective way—no matter how prudent a manufacturer or researcher may be—to prove there are no negative, long-term effects. This applies not only to pyruvate, but to a host of other supplements as well as drugs. So the fact that there are no known long-term negative effects associated with pyruvate usage doesn't mean some might not eventually show up.

To address this situation, it's recommended that you cycle your pyruvate intake. You could take it for three months, discontinue usage for four weeks, then go back on it for another three months, and so on. Or you could use it for six weeks, take a week off, go back on it for six weeks, etc.

"I think [taking pyruvate in cycles] is the safest way to go," says Dr. Stanko, "since I can't answer for the long-term toxicity. I think it's the safest way to go with any nutritional product, to tell you the truth. Even vitamins—like vitamin C. Take them for a reasonable period, then go off for a little bit."[41]

Again, all indications are that there are no adverse long-term effects from pyruvate supplementation; nevertheless, exercise caution and good judgment as suggested.

Dosage: How Much Is Enough?

According to Dr. Stanko, most of us consume about three-quarters to one gram of pyruvate a day in our normal diet—unless we drink red wine and eat red apples and cheeses in excess. Most fresh vegetables also have a little bit of pyruvate.

Since a gram a day isn't the optimum amount of pyruvate you want to be getting, Dr. Stanko advises, "You've really got to get it into your body through supplementation. It's the only way to do it. It's almost impossible to do it by changing your diet."

And how much pyruvate should one take daily in the form of dietary supplementation? Dr. Stanko claims that his studies have shown two to five grams of pyruvate is the optimal dosage, and that taking any more than that will not produce better results:

> You can take all you want—and I know there are body-builders out there taking this stuff now like you can't believe, and it does work. I took it to lift weights—it works. Runners are taking it—they can run farther. But once you get above five grams, you're just sort of wasting your time and money. We don't have any evidence that taking ten grams is bad for you. But we have absolutely all the evidence in the world that taking ten is no better than

taking five. So about five grams is your maximum recommended intake on pyruvate.[42]

However (and this may be the biggest "however" in the pyruvate phenomenon thus far), Dr. Stanko has never produced any documentation on these studies, despite the fact he's been engaged in a legal battle concerning patents and has been challenged to produce such documentation, which would greatly strengthen his case.

As of this writing, the public is left somewhat in limbo since no concrete scientific data regarding the precise pyruvate dosage levels that should be used has been made available. That being the case, individuals have to use a trial-and-error approach, keeping in mind that even Dr. Stanko himself has said: "In order for pyruvate to have its effect, the cell has to be maximized with pyruvate concentration."

The Beale Research Center in San Francisco recently completed a double-blind study on sixteen overweight women, average age of fifty, and found no measurable impact on fat loss from pyruvate supplementation at dosages under five grams.[43]

Perhaps it's only common sense that there's no way you could stipulate a set dosage that would be equally effective for everybody, because there are a lot of variables involved.

Pax Beale says that, generally speaking, the older you are, the better pyruvate seems to work, because your body loses pyruvate with age. You need to replenish what age has taken out; your need is greater. Another factor is how much fat you're carrying on your body—pyruvate seems to work better on fatter people. In addition to age and body fat, the person's physical size is a factor—a 100-pound housewife will need less pyruvate than a 250-pound football player. It's also important to consider what a person is trying to accomplish with pyruvate supplementation. For all these reasons Beale maintains that you can't project that a person should take a certain amount. And experience seems to indicate that some people need to take more than others.

"I've taken pyruvate in a wide variety of dosages," he says, "everything from two to five grams a day to eighteen grams. In a sense, I've used my body as a testing machine. My recommendation is that you start with a higher dosage until you saturate your body and get the response you want, then back off to a maintenance level. But I would not exceed twelve grams a day."[44]

The interesting thing about pyruvate is that apparently you can't take too much. Once you take in the amount of pyruvate your system can absorb and use, any excess pyruvate will simply end up being excreted from the body. That's another reason why you may initially want to start at a higher dosage to ensure you're getting results, and then cut back on the amount.

Manufacture and Availability of Pyruvate

Pyruvate is now manufactured by several companies and is available in capsule and powder form, as well as in bars and drinks. Methods of production, which require technical expertise and sophisticated equipment, include biofermentation and biochemical synthesis.

Pyruvate is made from pyruvic acid, the active ingredient, which is commercially combined with a mineral such as calcium or sodium to form a "salt" of pyruvic acid or, in lay terms, pyruvate. Pyruvate salt compounds would include calcium, sodium, potassium, magnesium and zinc pyruvate. It appears that calcium, magnesium and zinc pyruvate hold the most promise for the future. Sodium has two major disadvantages—it causes water retention and can lead to hypertension and heart disease. Potassium's disadvantage is that it presents serious manufacturing problems.

Pyruvic acid can also be combined with an amino acid or other compounds. Pyruvylglycene is the favored alternative as it appears to be a more efficient source of the active ingredient, pyruvate, and overcomes the nausea problem at high doses. Extensive research has been done on pyruvylglycene and patents exist on its manufacturing process. The major problem is that no one has yet conceived of a way to produce it economically.

13

THE FUTURE PROSPECTS

Clearly, more research is needed, over a greater span of years and usage, for us to fully understand the depth and scope of the health and metabolic benefits of pyruvate. Already pyruvate offers wonderful possibilities as a dietary supplement for athletes. What athlete wouldn't be interested in a supplement that augmented the beneficial effects of exercise and offered increased muscle glycogen, increased fat loss and increased endurance?

More research is also needed on the effects of pyruvate on non-obese, highly trained men and women. Thus far, almost all pyruvate studies have been done on "normal" people, many of them overweight and unfit, or on animals. It would be simple to do a pyruvate study with Olympic-caliber athletes such as distance runners, swimmers or cyclists, to ascertain the endurance effects of supplementing with pyruvate.

Of course, one of the most exciting things about pyruvate is that it's an equal-opportunity benefactor, providing a myriad of benefits for people regardless of their health or exercise levels. Indeed, for an athlete the greatest benefit of pyruvate may be to simply run faster in a race or look better in a physique competition. But reducing obesity, controlling diabetes and hyperlipidemia, improving cardiac efficiency and function, inhibiting free radical production and all its implications—these are the important and relevant benefits as far as the masses are concerned.

Thus it can be said that pyruvate is a supplement for everyone, and what the future holds for this exciting nutraceutical, if we can indeed call it that, seems open-endedly positive.

Animal Application

Pyruvate has been extensively tested on animals, and its many benefits make it ideally suited as a feed additive.[45] It could be used as a dietary supplement for pets or to promote lean body mass for a slaughter class of animals such as swine. A smaller market exists in the case of performance animals like race horses, where pyruvate supplementation could result in greater endurance and better performance.

It's not likely pyruvate would be added to the diets of animals such as cattle because the amount of pyruvate needed to produce the desired effect would be too great.

Synergistic Effects of Pyruvate

It seems certain that in the future we'll see some exciting results by combining pyruvate with other substances like phosphatidylserene or *Garcinia cambogia,* as already mentioned. Such combinations could result in a synergistic effect greater than the sum of the individual parts.

Current research with pyruvate combining has gone on at the University of Pittsburgh School of Medicine and Abbott-Ross Laboratories where they have focused on pyruvate combined with dihydroxyacetone (DHA). The Beale Research Center has studied combinations of pyruvate with protein powder and anticortisol agents for superior synergistic effect. The anticortisol agents are believed to reduce muscle degradation during anabolic or muscle-building activities, the net effect of which is more lean body mass.

Another synergistic effect already uncovered is that taking pyruvate with a sugared drink is a more effective way to get it into your system. Furthermore, patents held by Dr. Robert Cade and his associates at the University of Florida, based on extensive research they conducted on pyruvate, clearly show that pyruvate could improve electrolyte drinks. Despite the fact that the pyruvate patents of Dr. Cade and his associates have not been put into effect yet, there is no doubt that continuing research and experimentation will produce many other useful synergistic combinations involving pyruvate in the future.

CONCLUSION

It is valuable to remember that pyruvate doesn't simply target one specific health or physiologic area such as fat loss or athletic performance. It affects the heart, cholesterol, free radicals, energy, diabetes control (for those who have that problem), endurance, and so many other aspects of our life and well-being. Where benefits are concerned, pyruvate is almost like a smorgasborg.

And if you happen to be a person for whom pyruvate does not work in one area, there's evidently a good chance it will work for you in another. In this regard, pyruvate takes on the mantle of becoming kind of a maintenance supplement, a "part-of-good-health" supplement, if you will.

Sure, pyruvate can help you lose those few extra pounds so you look better in a bathing suit on a beach, and it can help you perform better in that next 10K race you run.

Whether such things are going to significantly improve your health is questionable. But when the focus shifts to the heart, free radicals, possible disease prevention and all those other things you can talk about in discussing pyruvate, then you're truly dealing with preventive medicine. In that regard, pyruvate has the potential, it seems, to become a staple of our diet, almost like a one-a-day vitamin.

Yet, although it may seem that supplementing one's diet with pyruvate is a lot like taking vitamin C, or any other vitamin or mineral, there is one significant difference: With a lot of supplements, you don't necessarily get a noticeable effect, no gratification in terms of obvious benefits within the short term. But pyruvate supplementation—if the research and those who have used the product are to be believed—does give you noticeable benefits and gratification. Moreover, it can apparently do so in various areas such as greater energy and endurance, increased weight loss, greater feeling of well-being, etc. Even Dr. Stanko says, "When you go off of pyruvate—I've done it myself—you can't wait to get back on it because you feel a little bit less well when you're off of it." And no, in case anyone is wondering, pyruvate is not addictive.

Pax Beale addresses the issue of tangible benefits this way:

> Most people who might need to supplement their diet with vitamin A or C or iron—particularly vitamin A and C—the symptoms of not having enough of it aren't flagrantly obvious. And when you get enough of it, you don't see a tremendous difference in how you feel or look.

The research on vitamin A, C and iron is clear as to what the benefits are, even though you don't necessarily feel them. I guess with iron you can, because if you take iron supplements you no longer have "tired" blood, as they say, and so you have more energy. That's only true, of course, if you have an iron deficiency to start with.

But with pyruvate, the benefits are often something you can visually see, or actually feel. In my case, as my heart improved and the dead tissue regenerated and could no longer be detected by the best instruments of medical science, my breathing got better, I felt stronger, I no longer felt any chest discomfort, I didn't have to continue taking my chest medication—I could clearly observe the beneficial effects of pyruvate.

For those people who are interested in fat loss, or a lean body mass, you can see the difference when you're taking pyruvate. Or if you're an AIDS patient and you combine pyruvate supplementation with doctor-prescribed anabolic steroids as treatment of a catabolic disease (the damage or erosion of muscle common with AIDS patients), you can slow that process. You can see it.

So I think one difference between supplementing your diet with pyruvate and supplementing it with vitamins or minerals is that pyruvate can give you benefits that are tangible. A person on pyruvate who's lost weight can say, "I feel better, I look better, my self-esteem is higher." Most other supplements don't bring that type of gratification.[46]

One important respect in which pyruvate supplementation *is* similar to vitamin and mineral supplementation (other than the fact you ingest all of these supplements) is that the benefits are a known quantity based on the research. Beale explains:

There is no doubt that it's been medically proven that for good health and welfare there's a need at times to take products like vitamin A,C and iron. Pyruvate falls in that bracket. It's not in the bracket of some exotic Tibetan tree-trunk herb that supposedly does something for you, but nobody can tell you exactly what. It's not in that bracket. There's enough research on pyruvate to move it from the mystique category of "maybe it has some benefits" to putting it in the same nutritional ballpark as proven supplements with known benefits such as vitamins A,C and iron.[47]

The Last Word

It's interesting to note that Dr. Stanko emphasizes in his lectures that he makes no claims that pyruvate will either cure or prevent disease. All he talks about, he says, is "cause and effect with pyruvate," based on what research studies indicate.

Of course, since pyruvate is a nontoxic, natural substance, it can be argued that it's not exactly a matter of having to hammer down every last nail of proof to make a case that pyruvate definitely will produce this benefit or that benefit. Unlike the situation with many drugs we could mention, toxicity is not a factor with pyruvate—at least not as far as we know.

So, the picture is this: try the supplement, see if it produces the benefits researchers are talking about, and if it doesn't, you're no worse off than you were before—other than being out the expense of the supplement. But if it does work, isn't it worth it?

The truth is that nutritional science can't provide definitive answers about a lot of nutritional products because, as Dr. Stanko himself acknowledges, most nutritional products have not had double-blind, long-term-use studies done on them. And despite all the research done on pyruvate, it, too, falls into that category. However, Dr. Stanko feels this is not a major obstacle, providing that the people marketing nutritional products don't "make unethical claims" and "push the product for something that it isn't." He elaborates:

> As long as you're honest about what you're saying, and you're not making religiously goofy claims that this is going to make somebody live to be 190 with no disease, I think we can deal with the lack of long-term studies. I think honesty is the most important thing. If you as a consumer understand what you're taking, and the manufacturer's claims are within what we know scientifically, the lack of a long-term study is not going to be all that significant.
>
> At the same time I can't teach my medical students a fact until these long-term studies are done. And most nutritional products don't have them—that's the truth. I know that.
>
> We're not going to have the pyruvate long-term studies for ten to fifteen years. I don't know what's going to happen to you fifteen years from now if you take pyruvate. I don't know. I personally think as a scientist and a person, you'll be better off. But we also don't know the long-term

toxicity. We don't. I mean, we don't know the long-term toxicity of a lot of things. We can say that about almost every nutritional product—with the exception of those that have been used for many years.

But as long as we're aware of that, as long as we can understand what is going on, as long as we don't go out and say we're going to cure the world of every disease there is, we should be all right until such studies are available. We will do those studies. They take time to do. They take a lot of money to do. But we will make the effort to do those ongoing studies with time. I'm sure some of the people who are presently using pyruvate will be part of what we're saying about it fifteen years from now—you know, there are 20,000 people in Salt Lake City and 20,000 people in New York who have been taking pyruvate, and this is what happened fifteen years later.[48]

In the final analysis, how does the man who's probably done more research on pyruvate than anyone else sum up its benefits? During his Dallas lecture, Dr. Stanko offered this summation:

What I'm telling you now is what I know pyruvate can do—it makes your cells better off as far as energy is concerned. That's a guarantee. I mean, that's been proven. It probably decreases body fat, and a lot of us who have been taking it have found that, yes, it does. It also increases your ability to exercise, probably because of that energy.

Does it prevent cancer from happening? I don't know— I have no idea. It certainly looks good, though we'll never talk about it, claim it. That's just something that we know about it. If you read my scientific literature, yes, that data is there . . .

Is it going to slow down aging? I don't know. I don't think you can stop aging. Aging is part of a process. You certainly can live longer. You can be happier and healthier when you're older.

But what I would take pyruvate for is something we're not even going to claim—to prevent free radicals from being there. I think this is good for you. I really do. I think most scientists will agree with me on that. When you read the literature on the antioxidants, that's where the problem is—that they don't seem to work! Because all the big studies on antioxidants aren't showing a whole heck of a lot about anything. And consequently the antioxidant theory is now coming very much under fire . . .

Now what we're trying to do here is show that the antioxidant theory is correct. It's just not being looked at the right way, and you're not treating the problem the right way. You should treat with something such as an antioxidant, but also with something that inhibits the production of free radicals.

Another thing that I can almost guarantee you about pyruvate is that it will improve ischemic disease. I know I've got ischemic heart disease, and so do 90 percent of the people in this room. We know from studies in Vietnam that young soldiers in their twenties, when they died and autopsies were done, had ischemic disease. At that age! So we've got it. There's nothing we can do about it. I think pyruvate will be of benefit there—I really do. We have quite a bit of data to show that.

I've been asked: Would I take pyruvate for AIDS? Yes, I would. Absolutely I would. Would I take pyruvate for aging? Yes, I would. Would I claim it [as a benefit of pyruvate]? No, I wouldn't. But, yes, I think it might help someone who has AIDS. Some AIDS patients can have AIDS for ten years and nothing happens, and others with the disease seem to die in an hour. Those that have poor nutritional balance are probably those that do the worst. So I would say, yes, I'd take pyruvate for AIDS. I would take it with other supplements though. I don't think pyruvate is the total answer to AIDS. AIDS is a multi-component problem, and you probably need more than one nutrient.

And that's basically what I can tell you about pyruvate for sure. My personal feeling is, since it's a natural compound, it's in your body at all times, and it's in the food chain. . . .[49]

We can all fill in the rest of that sentence for ourselves: Why not supplement our diet with pyruvate, considering its long list of benefits on the one hand and its apparent safety on the other?

ENDNOTES

1. Stanko, R.T., Robertson, R.J., et al, "Enhanced leg-exercise endurance with a high-carbohydrate diet, DHA and pyruvate," *Journal of Applied Physiology* 69: 1651-1656, 1990.
2. Cortez, M.Y., Torgan, C.E., Brozinick, J.T., Miller, R.H., Ivy, J.L., "Effects of pyruvate and dihydroxyacetone consumption on the growth and metabolic state of obese Zucker rats," *American Journal of Clinical Nutrition* 53: 847-853, 1991.
3. Stanko, R.T., U.S. Patent 5,134,162. Method for lowering high blood cholesterol levels in hyperlipidemic animals.
4. Stanko, R.T., U.S. Patent 5,480,909. Method for inhibiting generation of free radicals.
5. Several studies and patents substantiate this claim—e.g., see 33 and 37 below.
6. Stanko, R.T., U.S. Patent 5,480,909. Method for inhibiting generation of free radicals.
7. Documentary film, *Lethal Medicine.* The Nature of Wellness. Glendale, CA. 1997.
8. Beale, Pax. 1997. Personal interview with author.
9. Ibid.
10. Ibid.
11. Stanko, R.T. Lecture, Sterling Health Marketing Group. Dallas, TX. 1997.
12. Ibid.
13. Ibid.
14. Ibid.
15. Ibid.
16. Stanko, R.T., Robertson, R.J., et al, "Enhancement of arm exercise endurance capacity with DHA and pyruvate," *Journal of Applied Physiology* 68:119-124, 1990.

17. Beale, personal interview.
18. Ibid.
19. Ibid.
20. Ibid.
21. Ibid.
22. Cade, R., Privette, M., et al, U.S. Patent 4,981,687. Compositions and methods for achieving improved physiological response to exercise.
23. *L.A. Weekly,* July 18-24 issue, 1997.
24. Stanko, R. T., lecture.
25. Stanko, R.T., Tietze, D.L., Arch, J.E., "Body composition, energy utilization and nitrogen metabolism with a severely restricted diet supplemented with pyruvate," *American Journal of Clinical Nutrition* 55: 771-775, 1992.
26. Beale, personal interview.
27. Stanko, lecture.
28. Ibid.
29. Ibid.
30. Ibid.
31. Ibid.
32. Ibid.
33. Stanko, R.T., Mullick, P., Clarke, M.R., et al, "Pyruvate inhibits growth of mammary adenocarcinoma 13762 in rats," *Cancer Research* 1994; 54: 1004-1007.
34. Stanko, lecture.
35. Ibid.
36. Stanko, R.T., U.S. Patent 4,874,790. Method for improving the glucose metabolism of an animal having diabetic tendencies.
37. Stanko, R.T., and Adibi, S.A., "Inhibition of lipid accumulation and enhancement of energy expenditure by the addition of pyruvate and dihydroxyacetone to a rat diet," *Metabolism* 1986; 35:182-186.
38. Miller, Robert, et al, U.S. Patent 5,508,308. Use of pyruvylglycene to treat ischemia/reperfusion injury following myocardial infarction.
39. Stanko, lecture.

40. Ibid.
41. None of the studies on pyruvate have shown adverse side effects at sensible dosages.
42. Stanko, lecture.
43. Beale Research Center study, 1996, pyruvate dosage and body composition.
44. Beale, personal interview.
45. Stanko, R.T., et al, "Reduction of carcass fat in swine with dietary addition of DHA and pyruvate," *Journal of Animal Science*, 1989.
46. Beale, personal interview.
47. Ibid.
48. Stanko, lecture.
49. Ibid.

ABOUT THE AUTHOR

David Prokop is a Los Angeles writer whose work has appeared in many health and fitness publications. To date he has had more than 500 magazine articles published. A lifelong athlete, he has held several national and world endurance records. Former editor of *Runner's World* and *Muscle & Fitness* magazines, he is now director of the American Sports College on the Internet.